SANDY K NUTRITION

HEALTH & LIFESTYLE QUEEN PODCAST

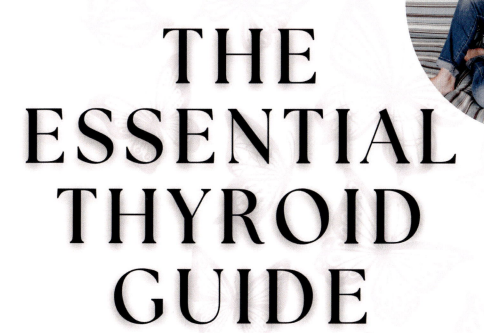

THE ESSENTIAL THYROID GUIDE

By Sandy Kruse

SANDY@SANDYKNUTRITION.CA

NOTES

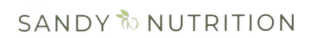
_____

_____

_____

_____

_____

_____

_____

_____

_____

_____

CONTENTS

SANDY NUTRITION

HEALTH & LIFESTYLE QUEEN PODCAST

NOTES

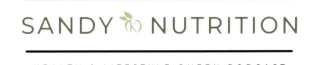

SANDY NUTRITION

HEALTH & LIFESTYLE QUEEN PODCAST

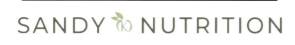

SANDY 🌿 NUTRITION

HEALTH & LIFESTYLE QUEEN PODCAST

Hello!

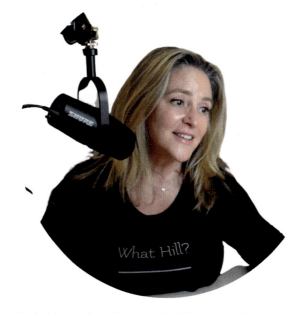

What Hill?

I am Sandy Kruse, host and creator of the popular _Sandy K Nutrition Health & Lifestyle Queen Podcast_, now at over 1.3 million downloads.

I am also a Registered Holistic Nutritionist, a Certified Metabolic Balance Coach, a Biohacker and an aging-well advocate at 54 years of age. I have taken certifications in Endocrinology and Hormones, Functional Lab Testing for Nutritionists and Peptides and Anti-aging. I hold a Bachelor's degree in English Literature, and at 49, graduated with a diploma in Holistic Nutrition from the Canadian School of Natural Nutrition.

I educate on alternative means for holistic health, wellness and preventative care, and share them with the world through my podcast and social media presence.

I believe all humans need a little of everything to be aligned in body, mind, and soul. Post-thyroidectomy due to thyroid cancer at 41, after many years of trying so many different methods of living and eating, I assert that balance is the key to living well, enjoying life, and living life well into those golden years – both happy and healthy.

I am working on my first book which speaks to balance in life by looking at all aspects of wellness to incorporate a little bit of science and a lot of soul.

DISCLAIMER: This guide is not medical advice and this is primarily written to educate on hypothyroidism. You must always see your practitioner for what's right for you, but please see the right practitioner who is trained in what your specific needs are. This is for educational purposes only.

Sandy Kruse

sandyknutrition.ca
sandykruse.ca
sandy@sandyknutrition.ca

NOTES

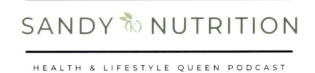

The Purpose of This Guide

This guide is not medical advice and is for educational purposes only.

I have a great deal of experience in thyroid health having lived without one since 2011, now living healthfully, optimally, without one, and have learned in hindsight how being proactive with thyroid health could have helped me. Now my insight, experience and education can help others.

I created this guide to educate you so you can work with your qualified practitioner to become a partner in your wellness journey, which is why I added a "Notes" page so that you can jot questions and your own symptoms for each section. *Remember this - no one knows or understands your own body as well as you do*, which is why understanding how things you do can affect thyroid and why you may feel a certain way is so important. Symptoms matter.

All in the name of health and wellness. I feel you and I'm with you. Many blessings to you on your thyroid journey.

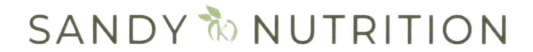

SANDY 🌿 NUTRITION

HEALTH & LIFESTYLE QUEEN PODCAST

sandy@sandyknutrition.ca

NOTES

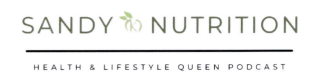

_____

_____

_____

_____

_____

_____

_____

_____

_____

_____

What Does the Thyroid Do - Why is it SO Important?

1
_____

It regulates the body's metabolic rate

2
_____

It plays a role in controlling heart, muscle and digestive function, brain development and bone maintenance.

This little butterfly-shaped gland in your neck has a role in every important function within your body. It controls if you're hot, if you're cold, if you can sleep or not, if you're happy, or sad, if you're temperamental or submissive, if you're thin or if you're fat and so much more.

This tiny little organ is a vital organ to life and we must care for it, and keep it if we can because no pill can control thyroid function the same as a healthy thyroid can.

NOTES

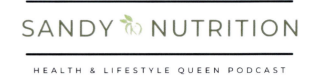

Nodules and Goiter

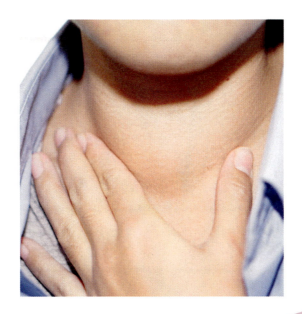

Nodules: An abnormal growth of cells, usually benign, within your thyroid gland - common

Goiter: A lump, swelling or enlargment of the thyroid

Possible Causes:
- Iodine deficiency
- Low vitamin D levels doi: 10.5144/0256-4947.2022.83
- Family history
- Increasing age
- Anemia
- Obesity

Possible Causes:
- Iodine deficiency
- Iodine excess (rare)
- Hashimoto's or Grave's
- Thyroiditis (inflammation of the thyroid)
- Nodules
- Estrogen dominance

NOTES

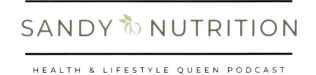

What is Hyperthyroidism?

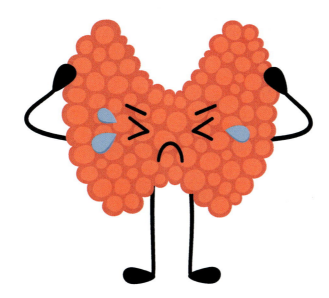

The thyroid gland makes too much thyroid hormone, also referred to as overactive thyroid, and yes, this means your TSH is TOO low or suppressed... NOT too high.
(I know this can be confusing)

Multiple factors can lead to this including:
- Grave's Disease
- Genetics
- Nutritional deficiencies
- Gut issues
- Poor lifestyle

NOTES

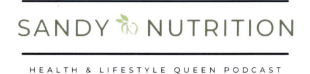

SANDY NUTRITION

HEALTH & LIFESTYLE QUEEN PODCAST

_____

_____

_____

_____

_____

_____

_____

_____

_____

_____

Checklist of Symptoms/Risks of Hyperthyroidism

Your TSH is at the lower end of the range - Below 0.35

Not all symptoms are felt by all * Indicates they may also menopause symptoms!**

- [ ] Anxiety***
- [ ] Weight loss
- [ ] Weight gain from nervous overeating***
- [ ] Difficulty sleeping***
- [ ] Heart palpitations***
- [ ] Shakiness/jitters
- [ ] Feeling hot/heat intolerance***
- [ ] Racing mind***
- [ ] Anger/temper***
- [ ] ADHD symptoms***
- [ ] Diarrhea
- [ ] Dry eyes/thyroid eye disease***
- [ ] Goiter
- [ ] Heart disorders***
- [ ] Osteoporosis***
- [ ] Graves autoimmune disease
- [ ] Above 98.2 F for several days using the Barnes Basal Temperature Test
- [ ] Hair loss***

NOTES

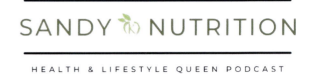

_____

_____

_____

_____

_____

_____

_____

_____

_____

_____

What is Hypothyroidism?

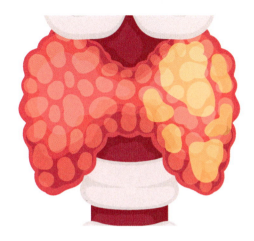

The thyroid gland does not make enough thyroid hormone, also referred to as underactive thyroid, and yes, this means your TSH is TOO high...NOT too low.
(I know this can be confusing)

Multiple factors can lead to this including:
- Hashimoto's Disease
- Genetics
- Nutritional deficiencies
- Gut issues
- Poor lifestyle

NOTES

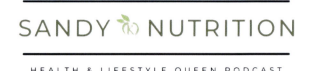

_____

_____

_____

_____

_____

_____

_____

_____

_____

_____

Checklist of Symptoms/Risks of Hypothyroidism

Your TSH is at the higher end of the range (some experience some symptoms above a 2 TSH even though range goes to 5)

Not all symptoms are felt by all * Indicates they may also menopause symptoms!**

☐ Dry skin, dry eyes***

☐ Puffy face

☐ Wrinkles***

☐ Depression***

☐ High cholesterol***

☐ Low energy & vitality***

☐ Feeling cold

☐ Migraine/headaches***

☐ Focus/memory issues***

☐ Heavy periods***

☐ Fertility issues***

☐ Muscle weakness***

☐ Achey joints***

☐ Brittle nails***

☐ High blood pressure***

☐ Hypoglycaemia***

☐ Outer 3rd of eyebrows missing

☐ Weight gain***

☐ Goiter

☐ Infections that take long to heal or won't heal

☐ Hashimoto's autoimmune disease

☐ Below 97.6 F for several days using the Barnes Basal Temperature Test

☐ Hair loss***

☐ Slow/weak pulse

☐ Macular degeneration

☐ Numbness/nerve issues

☐ Insulin resistance***

Hypo Thyroidism

NOTES

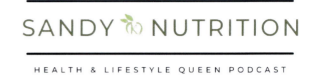

_____

_____

_____

_____

_____

_____

_____

_____

_____

_____

Thyroid Labs and what they mean (*** means they're most important to ask for!)   this is a sheet for you to print off   note there are many nutrients to support thyroid health not mentioned here

- **TSH** - This is the most common thyroid measurement, thyrotropin, and most doctors will do this without question. This is "Thyroid Stimulating Hormone" and isn't an actual thyroid hormone measurement! It is the hormone from your pituitary gland to signal to the thyroid to make hormones. When TSH is high, this means you're hypothyroid and your thyroid is underactive. Low TSH means hyperthyroid and the thyroid is overactive. Most people feel best between a 1-2 TSH, but the range can be from 0.35-5.0! ***

- **Free T4** - Approximately 80% of what the thyroid produces is T4 or thyroxine. This is the inactive form of thyroid hormone that must be converted to the active form to do it's work within the body. We want to see the "free" and unbound amount here. If you're with an endocrinologist, they will likely check this regularly. Your family physician will only check this if they feel it's necessary.***

- **Free T3** - Approximately 20% of what the thyroid produces is T3 or triiodothyronine and this is the active form the body needs to function properly. Again, we need to see the "free" and unbound amount here. If you're with an endocrinologist, they will likely check this regularly. Your family physician will only check this if they feel it's necessary.***

- **Reverse T3** - This hormone, triiodothyronine, is a biologically inactive hormone and a by-product of T4 degradation. When elevated, this blocks the conversion of the inactive T4 to the active T3. High reverse T3 can be caused by several factors including high stress and hyperthyroidism. Fun Fact - did you know that this can be elevated from carbohydrate deprivation?

- **TRH** - Thyrotrophin-releasing hormone or thyroliberin is made within the hypothalamus and regulates the secretion of TSH. It also stimulates the production of the hormone, prolactin. This is not a common thyroid panel test performed.

- **TPOab** - antithyroid peroxidase antibodies. These are often elevated in Hashimoto's Thyroiditis which is an autoimmune condition responsible for approximately 80% of hypothyroid cases. Also elevated in Grave's Disease which is an autoimmune condition responsible for hyperthyroidism. Can also be elevated with thyroid cancer but only in 10-20% of cases.

- **TRAb** - specific antibodies used to diagnose Grave's Disease.

- **Thyroglobulin** - typically used for patients who have had thyroid cancer but also if elevated can indicate insufficient iodine for healthy thyroid function.

- **Thyroglobulin Antibodies** - for diagnosing thyroid autoimmune diseases

NOTES

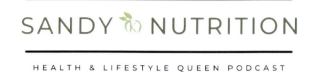
_____

_____

_____

_____

_____

_____

_____

_____

_____

_____

Thyroid Lab Ranges

(Note there maybe slight variances depending on male or female, age, pregancy and ranges vary as do metrics used so follow ranges for your country and look to be in the mid range for optimal)

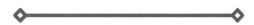

- **TSH:**
  - **0.35-5.00 mIU/L, 0.4 to 4.0 mIU/L**
- **Free T4:**
  - **11-23 pmol/L, 7.5 - 19.4 ng/L**
- **Free T3:**
  - **3.4-5.9 pmol/L, 2.3 – 4.1 pg/mL**
- **Reverse T3:**
  - **9.2-24.1 ng/dl**
- **TRH - 5-25 U/ml**
- **Anti-TPO - <30 IU/ml**
- **TPOAb - <9 IU/mL**
- **TRAb - 0 - 0.9 IU/L**
- **Thyroglobulin - 3-40 ng/mL - almost undetectable if you've had thyroid removed**
- **Thyroglobulin Antibody (TgAb) - <116 IU/mL**

- I am adding Vitamin D in because of it's importance to thyroid health & overall health. We **must** sit in optimal range of Vitamin D, not the lower ranges or lower end of normal. The range is **76-250 nmol/L but try to get over 150 nmol/L in Canada. Other range measurements are 20-40 ng/mL**

NOTES

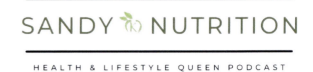

_____

_____

_____

_____

_____

_____

_____

_____

_____

_____

Thyroid Medications

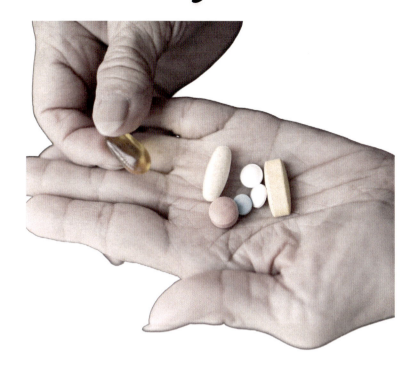

Let me say this loud and clear so the people in the back can hear - Synthroid or T4-only medications more often than not leave patients with lingering symptoms (go to Symptoms section for hypothyroid for these symptoms). See video for more detail on this.

- Other thyroid medications include (this may not be a comprehensive list for all countries):
- <u>Tirosint</u> (T4 only)
- <u>Tirosint-Sol</u> (T4 only)
- <u>Nature-throid</u> (T4 + T3 NDT)
- <u>Armour thyroid</u> (T4 + T3 NDT)
- <u>NP thyroid</u> (T4 + T3 NDT)
- <u>Cytomel</u> (T3 only)
- <u>Liothyronine</u> (T3 only)
- <u>Compounded T4 and T3 thyroid medication</u> (T4 + T3 non-NDT) - Ask the pharmacist what ingredients are used in compounded medications. I tried compounded thyroid medications once, and they used an ingredient that was a derivative of pine. I am allergic to pine, and found out the hard way. Be sure to ask questions.

Mostly every drug you take will result in some nutrient depletion. For more speak to your pharmacist, not your doctor, about medication interactions or go to drugs.com and use their Interactions Checker. Most thyroid medications are best taken on an empty stomach away from calcium

NOTES

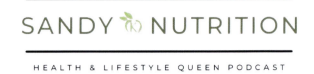

Toxins to Avoid

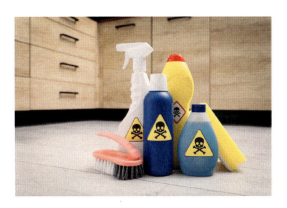

Ever feel like you're doing everything right
but you still don't feel well?
Often we forget about what we put on our skin,
our bodies, or use in or around our homes.
It's a huge contributing factor

Triclosan is in antibacterial soaps, cleaning products & many personal care products & structurally "looks" like T4 & can interfere with the function of T4

Pesticides & Herbicides are in our food & all around us increase risk of hypothyroidism

Parabens in makeup, creams & personal care products overall hormone disruptors

Phthalates in vinyl, plastics & personal care products associated with thyroid hormone disruption (& all other hormones too!)

NOTES

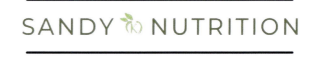

_____

_____

_____

_____

_____

_____

_____

_____

_____

_____

A Word About Halogens
(no one talks about this)

These are 6 Chemically Related Elements: fluorine (F), chlorine (Cl), bromine (Br), iodine (I) (#1 nutrient for your thyroid), and the radioactive elements astatine (At) and tennessine (Ts)

When you do not eat enough iodine-rich foods like fish, seafood, seaweed, eggs, etc, other halogens, most notably, chlorine and fluoride (fluorine is the element; fluoride is an ion or a compound which contains the fluoride ion) take up a "parking spot" in thyroid receptor as if they're iodine!

These chemically-similar compounds interfere with absorption of the actual nutrient the thyroid needs - IODINE!

What to do?

Work with a practitioner on various protocols to "push" out damaging halogens.
Eat iodine-rich foods.
Not a one-size-fits-all solution

NOTES

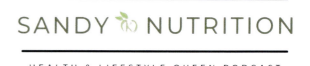

Importance of Detox

I have heard absurdities that detox is unnecessary & that our organs are designed to detox themselves. While that may have been true in the 1900's when assaults to our bodies were low, this couldn't be farther from the truth now in modern day society with constant assaults. For health optimization, a consistent approach preventing damage from these assaults is a great idea it isn't about buying a detox "box" off the shelf (major detoxes require working with an EXPERIENCED practitioner). Here are a few ideas...

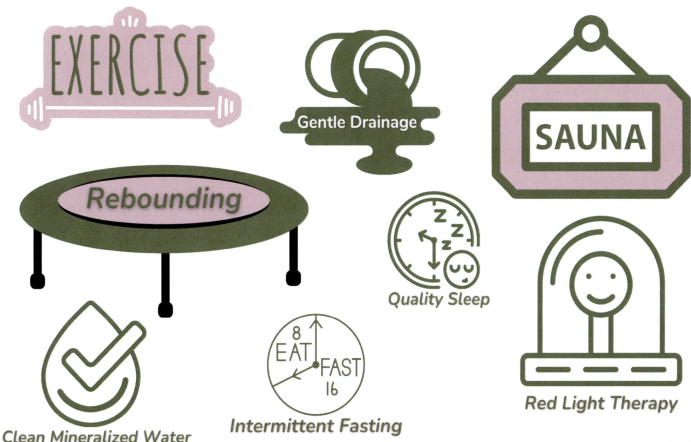

EXERCISE

Gentle Drainage

SAUNA

Rebounding

Quality Sleep

Clean Mineralized Water

Intermittent Fasting

Red Light Therapy

NOTES

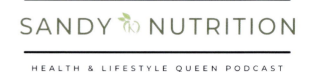

Factors that Affect Thyroid Function

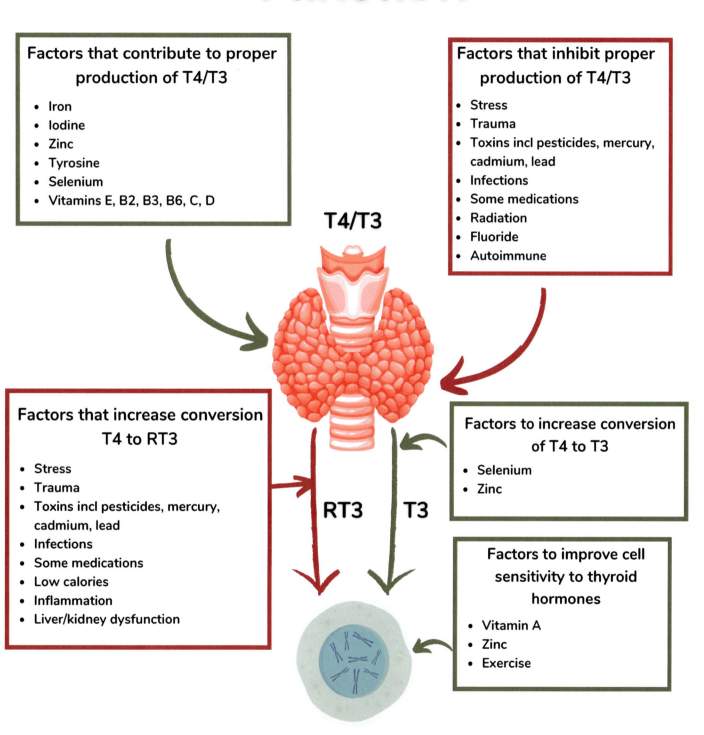

Factors that contribute to proper production of T4/T3

- Iron
- Iodine
- Zinc
- Tyrosine
- Selenium
- Vitamins E, B2, B3, B6, C, D

Factors that inhibit proper production of T4/T3

- Stress
- Trauma
- Toxins incl pesticides, mercury, cadmium, lead
- Infections
- Some medications
- Radiation
- Fluoride
- Autoimmune

T4/T3

Factors that increase conversion T4 to RT3

- Stress
- Trauma
- Toxins incl pesticides, mercury, cadmium, lead
- Infections
- Some medications
- Low calories
- Inflammation
- Liver/kidney dysfunction

Factors to increase conversion of T4 to T3

- Selenium
- Zinc

RT3   T3

Factors to improve cell sensitivity to thyroid hormones

- Vitamin A
- Zinc
- Exercise

This is the cell where T3 needs to do it's job

NOTES

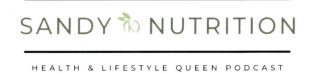

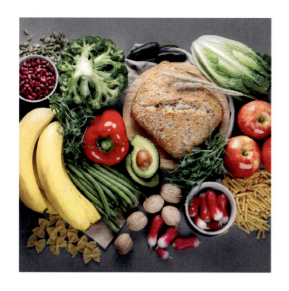

Food As Medicine to Support Thyroid Health

Here are some important points for thyroid health & to help you maintain & even lose weight - this is especially for those around menopause with thyroid dysfunction. We are all bioindividual. The main thing is to eat whole real foods, and focus on what feels good in your body.

I struggled to keep weight balanced since I had my thyroid removed in 2011 and even before it was removed. After the birth of my second child, I can now surmise that I had all the symptoms of postpartum thyroiditis that continued on and was never diagnosed.

The ONLY diet, and yes, diet, was my own Metabolic Balance program that helped me to lose fat, maintain muscle and bone. I will provide you with the most important rules for this program, and if you wish to do the actual program, get in touch with me. It is worth the investment, for I have never found a diet that "fixed" my metabolism so that my weight remained stable. In November 2022, I began my own program, lost 4% total body fat, and maintained it as I am writing this in February 2024.

Don't tell me a menopausal women without a thyroid has to gain weight...Can you imagine LOSING fat, maintaining muscle and actually improving bone mineral density at 53?

Maintaining a healthy weight & body composition is critical to overall health. It's not about being skinny. It's about being healthy. Obese isn't healthy & I won't sugar coat this. We cannot be healthy at every size...

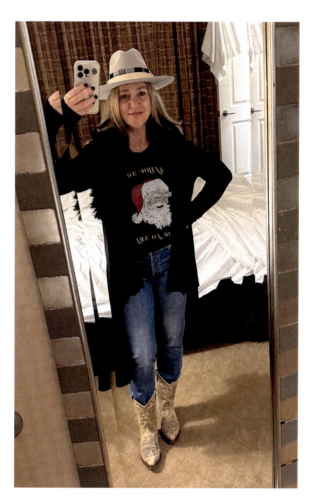

Make lasting changes

NOTES

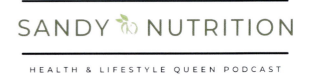
_____

_____

_____

_____

_____

_____

_____

_____

_____

_____

_____

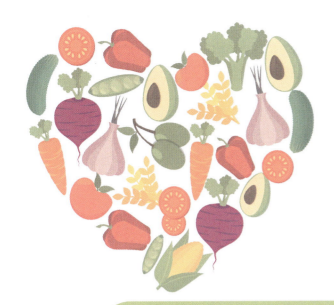

Golden Rules for Food

You've exhausted all efforts, medications don't work well, you're not getting better, and you haven't dialed in on what you're feeding your body.

You're forgetting the most important foundation of Food as Medicine. Most people don't realize just how important *how* you eat & *what* you eat is.

1. Every autoimmune condition is tied to the gut. At least for now, cut out gluten and dairy as these two food groups are tied to inflammation

2. Eat only whole, real foods that you cook at home with oils that are not inflammatory. Use only olive oil for cold (ie salads) and higher heat expeller pressed avocado oil or organic coconut oil for cooking.

3. Choose wisely - I have always said there are Good, Better, Best options. Everyone with some investigation can find foods that are better quality for better prices. Choose organic, pasture raised, grass fed whenever you can. Remember, these toxins, hormones & antibiotics affect thyroid.

4. Avoid all raw goitrogens including broccoli, cabbage, kale, Brussel sprouts, cauliflower, bok choy - you can find a comprehensive list online

NOTES

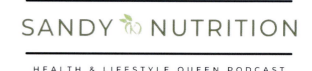

So You're Hypothyroid...
Foods 101

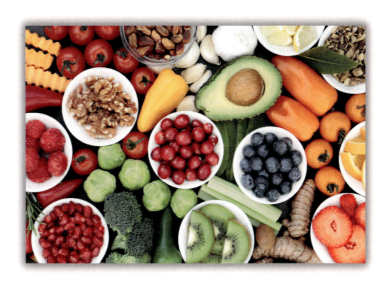

Too much soy can interfere with thyroid hormone medication so if you eat soy keep it 2 hours away from your meds. Even if not on thyroid meds, you might want to limit soy.

Cruciferous vegetables like cabbage, broccoli, cauliflower that are raw and in larger amounts can interfere with how your thyroid uses iodine & iodine is critical to healthy thyroid function.

Foods/Supplements to avoid within 2 hours of taking thyroid medications: calcium, iron, biotin, vitamin c, iodine.

Golden rule is always to eat whole real foods - as clean as possible. Use my 80/20 rule

NOTES

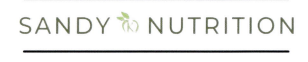

_____

_____

_____

_____

_____

_____

_____

_____

_____

_____

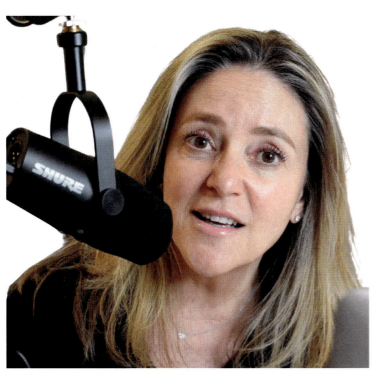

Golden Rules of Fat Loss At Menopause

1. Eat three meals a day, ZERO snacks
2. Five hour break between each meal
3. Ensure each meal lasts no longer than one hour
4. Begin every meal with two bites of protein
5. Don't eat past 8 pm
6. Drink water, but with every glass add a pinch of QUALITY mineralized sea salt like Celtic or Redmond sublingually under your tongue (put those darn 2 litre bottles away!!!)
7. Eat one apple everyday immediately after a meal
8. Try not to mix proteins & have only one protein at every meal
9. Choose movement that you align with, but move everyday, multiple times a day even if in just shorter bursts
10. Sleep well & prioritize your sleep
11. While we can't eliminate stress, we can mitigate effects of stress on our bodies
12. Meditation - use NuCalm or BrainTap for a shortcut
13. Throw away your numbers-only scale & get a body composition scale & track important trends like muscle, bone, visceral fat, total body fat
14. Be cognizant of issues with insulin resistance at menopause and take a glucose stabilizer if necessary. There is a clear connection between thyroid dysfunction and insulin resistance and lowering estrogen at menopause can make it even worse.

NOTES

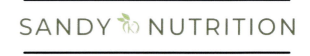

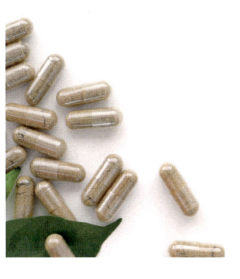

My Favourite Supplements

Go to myvitaminscore.com and use SANDYK for 25% off to assess your individual nutrient needs.
I do not believe in multivitamins except in specific situations.

I am not YOUR nutritionist. Supplements aren't a one-size fits all so work with your own practitioner (not family doctors as they're NOT educated in supplementation)

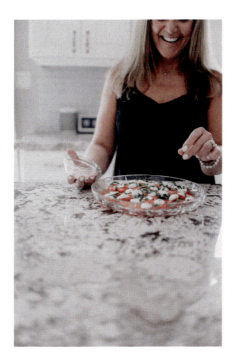

If you wish to consult with me get in touch

NOTES

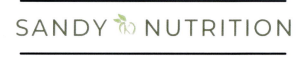
_____

_____

_____

_____

_____

_____

_____

_____

_____

_____

Thyroid Health & Spiritual Connection

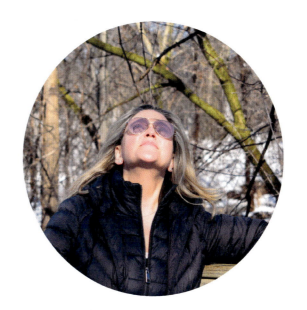

For every ailment, repeating accidents, pain, there is a connection to your body and what it's trying to telling you.

We cannot separate our spirit to our body's symptoms. It's a big miss in science maybe because it's too difficult to prove through studies.

But when you know you know. And when you start to uncover the emotional side, it can help you heal.

The throat chakra is considered the gateway between the mind and the body. The thyroid governs this area. This is the area of our personal power and self expression.

Have you felt in your life that you couldn't speak your truth? I'll give you an example here. I had loving parents, grew up in a healthy environment and had a healthy childhood. I also grew up in an environment where we weren't allowed to "talk back" or say no or really speak what was on our mind. I am a creative & expressive person so this affected me.

NOTES

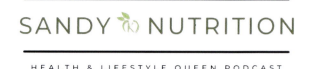

Critical Thinking Connecting Emotion To Thyroid Health

Louise L. Hay *You can Heal Your Life*
- Humiliation
- I never get to do what I want to do
- When is it my turn?

In the book <u>Messages From the Body</u> by Michael J. Lincoln there is a belief that those with thyroid disease have no right to express who they are, to develop, to put out and apply their creativity to succeed. This resonates with me so so much

Underactive:
- Feeling stuck
- Emotional hibernation
- Unexpressed resentment and frustration

Overactive:
- Not prioritizing your own life
- Always outward
- External validation

NOTES

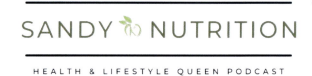

SANDY NUTRITION

HEALTH & LIFESTYLE QUEEN PODCAST

sandy@sandyknutrition.ca

Podcast Resources on Thyroid and Healing the Body

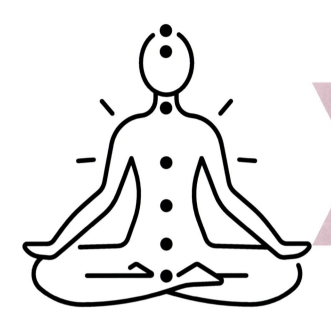

**Healing takes time and patience.
Sandy K Nutrition
Health& Lifestyle Queen
Podcast**

Episode 24 - Solo episode talking about the Biology of Belief by Dr. Bruce Lipton
Episode 44 - Podcast on thyroid with Dr. Lisa Koche
Episode 64 - Generational trauma with Mark Wolynn
Episode 66 - Resynchronize the body to heal itself
Episode 91 - Thyroid solo episode
Episode 136 - Thyroid with Dr. Lauren Bramley
Episode 141 - Theta Healing
Episode 142 - Limiting beliefs
Episode 152 - Braintap & your higher self
Episode 154 - The Sedona Method
Episode 158 - The Body Code with Dr. Bradley Nelson
Episode 192 - We can heal ourselves with Julia Cannon
Episode 202 - NuCalm for sleep and stress

Note that all episodes can be found on whichever podcast platform you listen on

NOTES

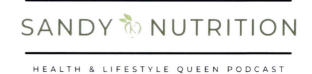

HEALTH & LIFESTYLE QUEEN PODCAST

Your Doctor Won't Test More than TSH - Now What?

It is essential to find a physician who will partner and advocate for your best health. If you have trouble finding this, keep interviewing doctors as there are some great ones there to support us. Sometimes our physicians can't do certain tests due to restrictions. In this case, there are numerous options to get proper testing in North America. I will note some below.

Ontario, Manitoba, Quebec, Canada:
bloodtestscanada.com

WORLDWIDE:
ZRT LABS

One of my personal favourite home blood test kits is from SiPhoxHealth.com use code SANDYK for a discount available in all of North America soon to expand

If you're a perimenopausal or menopausal woman, I suggest also checking diurnal cortisol & other sex hormones using dried urine with The Dutch Test which should be available internationally. Use my code SKN100 for $100 off. If your goal is to go on hormones, work with a doctor who understands the Dutch. If your goal is to use food and supplementation, you can book a consult with me.

51

NOTES

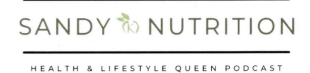

SANDY NUTRITION
HEALTH & LIFESTYLE QUEEN PODCAST

Thank-you!

It's my life's work to reach as many people to say that we can do so much with a little bit of patience & learning, to optimize our health.

I am truly grateful for my first "hard copy" creation to help others achieve wellness on their thyroid journey.
Please share my podcast with as many people to learn on many different modalies to be preventative and proactive with our wellness & look out for my book coming in 2024.

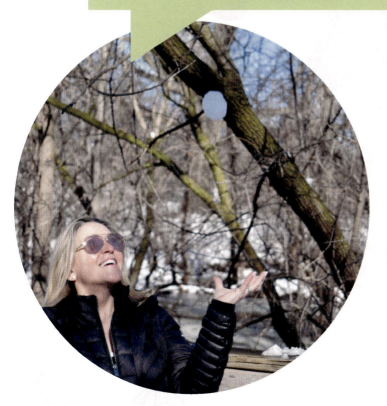

Contact:

sandykruse.ca
sandyknutrition.ca
sandy@sandyknutrition.ca

Follow Me:
Sandy K Nutrition on all the socials & podcasting platforms